C000133420

The Little
Book of
Chakras

The Little
Book of
Chakras

Balance your subtle energy for
health, vitality, and harmony

Patricia Mercier

An Hachette UK Company
www.hachette.co.uk

First published in Great Britain
in 2017 by Gaia, a division of
Octopus Publishing Group Ltd
Carmelite House
50 Victoria Embankment
London EC4Y 0DZ
www.octopusbooks.co.uk
www.octopusbooksusa.com

Distributed in the US by
Hachette Book Group
1290 Avenue of the Americas
4th and 5th Floors
New York, NY 10020

Distributed in Canada by
Canadian Manda Group
664 Annette St.
Toronto, Ontario
Canada M6S 2C8

ISBN 978-1-85675-370-8

A CIP catalog record for this book
is available from the British Library.

Printed and bound in China

10 9 8 7 6 5 4 3

Commissioning Editor
  Leanne Bryan
Editor Pollyanna Poulter
Art Director Juliette Norsworthy
Designer Rosamund Saunders
Illustrator Abigail Read
Senior Production Controller
  Allison Gonsalves

Disclaimers

All reasonable care has been taken
in the preparation of this book
but the information it contains is
not intended to take the place of
treatment by a qualified health or
medical practitioner.

Essential oils should not be used
for children under 12. If you
are pregnant, seek the advice of
a qualified aromatherapist. For
sensitive skin, do a skin test first.
Never ingest essential oils.

Contents

Introduction

The Sanskrit word "chakra" translates as "wheel" or "disk." Knowledge of chakras stems from the Upanishads (sacred Sanskrit texts), dating from 600 B.C.E., as well as having been transmitted orally by guru to student. Chakras are energetic centers in the subtle body, comprised of the mind and vital energies. They are depicted as lotus blossoms of color that progress from the Base Chakra to the Crown Chakra, with resonances that are similar to the colored light of rainbows.

The lotus is the national flower of India; it grows in muddy rivers, pushes up through the waters, blossoms in sunlight, seeds, and recycles itself, in much the same way we do. We are born in ignorance of our life-path, push through the emotions and setbacks that we encounter, and eventually flower in the full spirit of our excellence and potential, before passing on to the unknown.

In this book you will find practical ways to care for and nourish your chakras. Each activity takes just five or ten minutes to fit into your busy day on a regular basis.

Yoga and mindful exercise, coupled with self-improvement and relaxation techniques, have become popular in recent times because mind, body, and that essence sometimes called Spirit are intimately connected. This little book shares the energy teachings and wisdom that link these elements together.

I invite you to come on an exploration with me and to deepen your potential of personal development and mindfulness. By becoming aware of your chakras, you will learn to fully relax, heighten your consciousness, and improve your health and wellness.

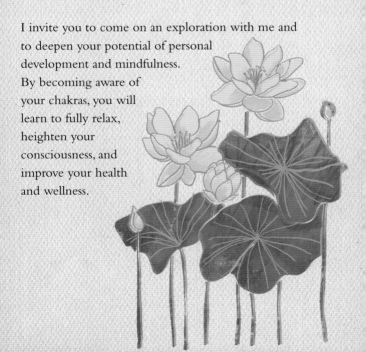

What are Chakras?

The chakras are vortices of subtle energy within the human aura—an electromagnetic field of varying vibrational frequencies often called our Luminous Body. Traditionally there are seven principal chakras—the Base Chakra, the Sacral Chakra, the Solar Plexus Chakra, the Heart Chakra, the Throat Chakra, the Brow Chakra, and the Crown Chakra— with a number of minor chakras also being mentioned in sacred texts originating in India.

In this book we are focusing on the seven main chakras, plus the newly developing chakras. These "higher-energy" chakras are the Earth Star and Hara Chakras and the celestial trio of the Causal, Soul Star, and Stellar Gateway Chakras.

Through these chakras flows incoming information that is of great benefit to our health, especially in stimulating and fine-tuning the actions of the endocrine glands and major body organs. These glands produce hormones, which in turn affect the whole body, ideally bringing about a balanced state of health and mind. Mystics and yogis (those who are proficient at yoga) know that without

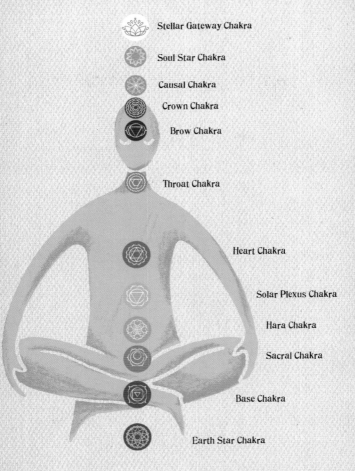

Stellar Gateway Chakra

Soul Star Chakra

Causal Chakra

Crown Chakra

Brow Chakra

Throat Chakra

Heart Chakra

Solar Plexus Chakra

Hara Chakra

Sacral Chakra

Base Chakra

Earth Star Chakra

the flow of subtle chakra energies, which are not as yet scientifically explained, we could not live. They are our vital links to the "Web of Life on Earth" (*see* page 70), drawing sustenance from a great cosmic energy field that enervates our personal auric field, chakras, and physical body.

By bridging traditional practice and cutting-edge research, this book shows that you do not have to practice super-difficult yoga asanas (postures) or lengthy meditations. It makes sense to love and care for your chakras in an accessible and regular way—as an "energy medicine"—to realize your full potential and express it in the world. Simple steps to clear the clutter from your mind and home, and to tune into what the natural world and your body are telling you, can increase vital pranic energy, our life-force. Ways to calm or tonify yourself through gentle movement, relaxation techniques, crystals (*see* page 60), and essential oils (*see* page 82) can all help to bring the chakras, mind, and body into balance, by boosting levels of the life-force, prana.

In addition, because urban areas are becoming increasingly chemically and electromagnetically toxic, you can help to reduce the stresses this causes to the body by choosing to live mindfully.

1
Base Chakra:
Grounding

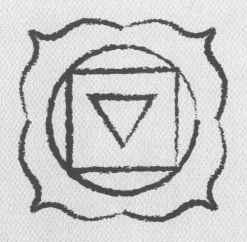

The Base Chakra—Muladhara

Grounding, deepening,
connecting to the environment.

- **Traditional meaning:** the root of Kundalini (*see* page 28); the four lotus petals represent forms of blissful joy.

- **Color:** resonates with red light frequencies.

- **Yantra (symbol):** four lotus petals, a yellow square (Earth), downward pointing red triangle (female energy), a lingam (phallic male energy), and an elephant with seven trunks (strength, the seven chakras and seven constituents that support the body).

- **Essential oils:** patchouli or myrrh to balance; cedarwood to cleanse.

- **Element:** sustained by the natural element of Earth.

- **Physical action:** sexuality.

- **Mental action:** brings stability.

- **Beneficial yoga asanas:** Virabhadrasana 1 (warrior), Trikonasana (triangle).

Located within the aura (our unique energy field), near the perineum, the Base Chakra establishes us upon the Earth, as it is very active in the first seven years of life, conveying into the body all the delicate energies and cosmic encodements required for growth. As we develop beyond puberty, this chakra stimulates the endocrine glands of the sexual organs, channeling energies into our reproductive system. It is closely connected with the Earth Star Chakra (*see* page 86).

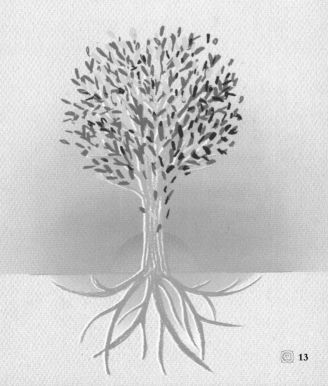

Balance the Base Chakra

Does your body feel ill at ease? An unbalanced Base Chakra suggests that the basic needs of the body are not being met. An indicator is that the spine, legs, testes, and blood-cell rejuvenation may be affected. This can result in a compromised metabolism— "the couch-potato effect"—and in increased weight. Key life-path issues concern sexuality, lust, obsessions, and being overly materialistic.

Excessive energy (when the chakra spins too fast) can lead to aggression, sexual neuroses, or dominating egotism.

Deficient energy (slow chakra spin) indicates lack of confidence, low will power, depression, lack of interest in sex, and lack of grounding.

There are numerous ways to bring balance to this chakra, as described in the five- and ten-minute practices and inspirations on the following pages, all helping us to be trusting of others and in touch with joyful emotions.

Balancing this chakra by grounding either excessive or low lethargic energy through inner intention and visualization or physical activity supports your core, bringing strength and resilience (for grounding visualization *see* pages 18–19).

Affirmation: "I seek balance and harmony in my life."

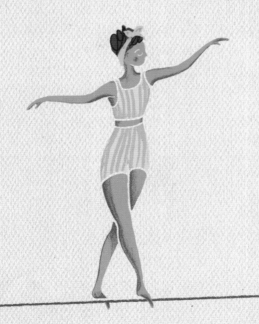

Activity: Relax and Refresh
(10 minutes)

This deep relaxation technique recharges all your chakras, releases mind stresses, and relaxes the body. You can do it every day if you wish, but first ensure that you will not be disturbed and that you have switched off any electronic devices.

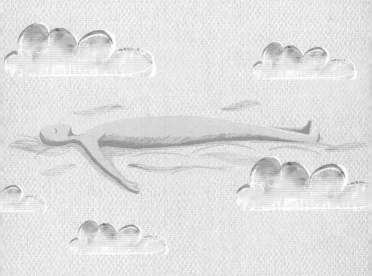

- Lie down on your back (in Savasana, the relaxation pose), somewhere warm and comfortable, but don't go to sleep.

- Close your eyes and take three deep breaths, releasing tension on the out-breath.

- Breathe normally and start to journey through your body, beginning with your right foot and working up the right leg to your hip, relaxing each part, muscle by muscle.

- Repeat with your left foot, leg, and hip.

- Relax your buttocks, sexual organs, pelvis, and lower back.

- Feel a wave of relaxation rippling up the front of your body as your spine "softens" and sinks down.

- Now relax your neck, and feel your arms and hands becoming limp and heavy.

- Finally, relax your jaw, smooth the muscles of your face, and let the activity in your brain slow down.

- When you want to finish (sometimes you might like to take up to 20 or 30 minutes), gently move each part of your body in turn and slowly sit up.

Activity: Ground the Chakras
(5 minutes)

This little visualization helps you to relax and feel subtle energies.

- Take time out to stand comfortably, or sit on a straight-backed chair. Close your eyes.

- Deepen your breathing; with every breath, breathe in calmness, exhale stress. When you are really calm, continue with the exercise, breathing normally.

- **Imagine:** "I am the link between Earth and sky. The nature of my consciousness sends roots through the soles of my feet, deep into the Earth, sensing my connection to nature.

  "I feel my roots extending to a crystal in the Earth's center, and immediately a vibrant burst of light shoots up from it into my body.

  "I feel this light pulsing through my body, chakras, and auric field, letting it ground, warm, relax, recharge, and heal me."

- Slowly open your eyes.

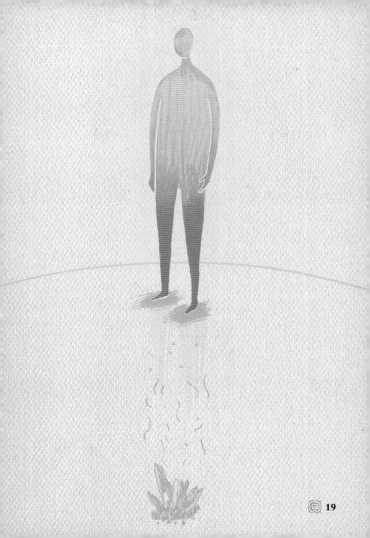

Activity: Color Breathing
(10 minutes)

An energizing, moving meditation or a deep relaxation for all the chakras—your choice.

- Take yourself outside or stand in front of an open window, eyes open. Breathe in each color, taking **three breaths for each chakra**.

- Touch the ground with your fingertips, honoring the life-giving Earth. Breathe in red light, feeling it re-energizing your legs and Base Chakra.

- Slowly standing up, draw energy up your body with your hands, resting them just below your navel while inhaling orange light, re-energizing your Sacral Chakra.

- Breathe yellow light into your Solar Plexus Chakra.

- Moving and swaying with your arms wide, inhale the life-giving, green light of nature into your Heart Chakra.

- Concentrating on your Throat Chakra, place your hands there, inhaling blue or turquoise light from the sky.

- Move your hands up to your Brow Chakra, holding them in a triangle shape, palms out, tips of the thumbs and forefingers touching. Breathe deep-blue light.

- Move the triangle of your hands onto your head. Breathe violet light into your Crown Chakra.

- Stretch your arms straight up, re-energizing your higher chakras with clear white-light breaths. Drawing your hands down the front of your body, now take just **one breath for each chakra**. Touch the ground with your fingertips and feel balanced.

- **To relax:** lie on your back, using the same breath colors without movements.

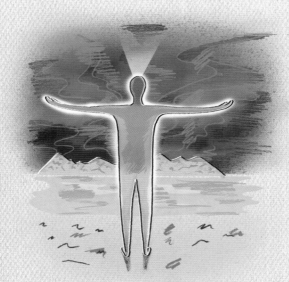

Activity: Reflexology Massage (5 minutes)

Reflexology is a complementary therapy that uses pressure on specific points on the feet and hands.

- Look at the illustrations and find your Base Chakra (red) point. Start either on the right hand or right foot, then repeat on the other hand or foot.

- Press firmly on the point and gently massage it, by rotating your thumb in a clockwise direction. If there is any discomfort on the point, press harder to disperse it.

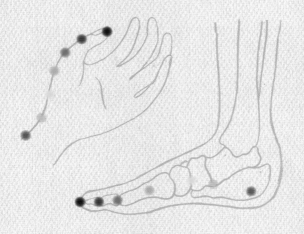

2
Sacral Chakra:
Pleasure

The Sacral Chakra—Svadisthana

Emotions, pleasure, relationships, creativity.

- **Traditional meaning:** "one's own abode"; the six open lotus petals represent creativity, sexual energies, and joy.

- **Color:** resonates with orange light frequencies.

- **Yantra:** six lotus petals, crescent moon (regeneration through female energy) and Makara—a mythic fish-tailed crocodile (sensuousness).

- **Essential oils:** sandalwood or ylang-ylang to balance; fennel to cleanse.

- **Element:** sustained by the natural element of Water.

- **Physical action:** balances sexuality.

- **Mental action:** harmonizes the emotions, joy, and relationships.

- **Beneficial yoga asana:** Parivrtta trikonasana (twisting triangle).

Located within the aura below the navel, the Sacral Chakra helps keep us well by constantly bringing subtle energy vibrations into our body. These are part of the electromagnetic field surrounding the planet and are compromised in our modern environment by a "fog" of electromagnetic pollution from items such as cellphones, microwave ovens, and medical X-ray procedures.

The Sacral Chakra is linked to the flow of liquids in our bodies. The glands that it stimulates are the adrenals, which are involved in responses to stress through the "fight or flight" reflex, when the body produces additional hormones. In a really desperate situation, this may save our life, but if this reflex is constantly triggered by little issues, it makes us prone to physical dysfunctions. This is a vital chakra to balance our levels of stress and, ultimately, our mental and bodily wellness.

The first two traditional chakras are our "recycling chakras": the Base and Sacral Chakras change negative emotional energies into power and light. They keep our aura clean, returning to Earth any "toxic waste" that the body cannot cope with.

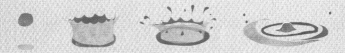

Balance the Sacral Chakra

Imbalances between the input and output of energies into the Sacral Chakra may lead to bladder and kidney disorders, circulatory problems, intestinal complaints, shallow breathing, migraines and reproductive system problems. Low energy levels go hand-in-hand with physical dysfunctions because of disturbances to the central nervous system, which are normally governed by inputs of beneficial energies through this chakra.

This is a very important chakra for women to balance. For centuries the repression of women has caused this energetic center—and others—to malfunction. Working regularly on all the chakras will help to release these types of ancestral or karmic blockages. (There is more about Karma—spiritual cause-and-effect—on page 91).

One of the symbols of the Sacral Chakra is the Moon, which is associated with the flow of water in nature, including body fluids. When water flows freely it becomes energized. Crying is nature's way to release tension—tears of joy have a different chemical content from those of sadness. Laughter feeds this pleasure chakra, eventually bringing great joy to our lives.

Excessive energy can lead to becoming overemotional, aggressive, manipulative, overindulgent, and sex-obsessed.

Deficient energy suggests oversensitivity, resentment, distrust, and guilt.

There are numerous ways to bring **balance** to this chakra, to be trusting of others and in touch with joyful emotions.

Affirmation: "I will approach whatever challenges life gives me with joy-filled actions."

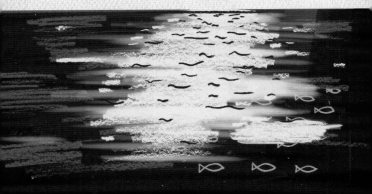

Kundalini Teachings

Kundalini is about sex: true or false?
The answer is both yes and no.

Traditionally, the aim of balancing the chakras is to arouse kundalini, which is depicted as a snake or as the Hindu goddess Shakti, who slumbers at the Base Chakra. Shakti ascends ecstatically through the chakra lotuses to couple with the Hindu god Shiva and eventually, on reaching the Crown Chakra, brings enlightenment.

Modern understandings describe kundalini as the great cosmic power that creates and sustains the universe, and therefore to move and increase that power throughout the body brings amplified wellness. Many great yogis have described the spontaneous awakening of kundalini. Various types of yoga—such as Shakti, Kundalini, and Tantric Yoga—have developed, all aiming to activate kundalini. Right intention, correct breathing, yoga asanas, and meditation are all central to its activation.

Fundamentally, at the Base Chakra, kundalini energy connects us to nature and enhances our sex life, while at the Sacral Chakra it increases our understanding of other people. At the Solar Plexus Chakra, it aids the assimilation of nourishment; at the Heart Chakra, it helps us to feel intense love; at the Throat Chakra, kundalini boosts the way we express ourselves; at the Brow Chakra, it enhances inner perceptions; and at the Crown Chakra, it takes us into altered states of consciousness.

Ultimately, the movement of kundalini brings a state of bliss that is momentarily experienced, as in orgasm, or is sustained as an ecstatic, prolonged, life-changing spiritual experience.

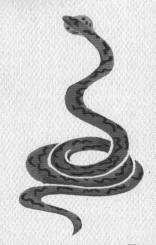

Activity: Relaxing Belly Breathing (5 minutes)

You can love your Sacral Chakra using the following technique.

- Kneel down or sit comfortably in a simple crossed-leg position (Sukhasana) or on a straight-backed chair.

- Rest your hands on your belly. Start by slowly inhaling and exhaling to a count of ten. Repeat three times, feeling your belly rise and fall with each breath.

- Now, with each incoming breath, push it down to the deepest part of your lungs—again you will feel your belly rise. Visualize channeling orange-colored light into each in-breath. When color-breathing in this way, it is often helpful to picture the colored light as a flower—in this instance, an orange marigold.

- Continue for up to five minutes and try to sense your Sacral Chakra. You may feel heat or vibration.

Activity: Sensing Chakras (10 minutes)

How are your chakras are spinning? You may intuitively know that they are too fast, too slow or in balance. Or you can use a method called Scanning.

Scanning uses an open palm, moving slowly over the front of your body or along the spine (of another person), without touching the body and within the auric field. You linger over each chakra to "scan" or sense it. You may feel warmth, vibration, or other sensations. This technique is very intuitive, so people generally interpret these feelings from inner perceptions and knowing.

Alternatively, you could check out your chakras with a pendulum (*see* page 50).

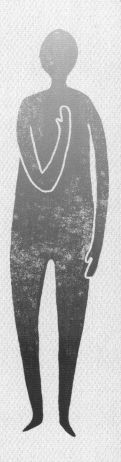

Activity: Giving Chakra Healing
(10 minutes)

**This technique is suitable for using either
on another person or on an animal.**

- Wash your hands. Turn off your cellphone/electrical
  devices and take a moment for both of you to become
  calm. Your friend (or animal) may sit or lie down.

- Hold your hands in the prayer position for a
  moment, then rub them together—this increases
  the healing frequencies.

- Ask if you may place your hands upon your friend's
  (the animal's) body, or whether they are more
  comfortable if you work in their auric field. Question
  inwardly which chakras need balancing or healing.

- Respectfully place your hands on or over their
  chakras and be still, radiating unconditional love
  to them for ten minutes. When you have finished,
  wash your hands again.

3
Solar Plexus Chakra: Fire

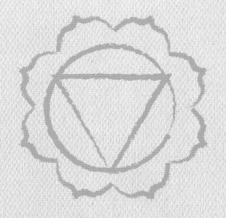

The Solar Plexus Chakra—
Manipura

Fire of metabolism, ego, zest for life.

- **Traditional meaning:** "jewel of the navel"; words on the ten lotus petals represent negative traits that are destroyed by fire.

- **Color:** resonates with yellow or golden light frequencies.

- **Yantra:** ten lotus petals, red triangle pointing down (Brahma/Vishnu/Shiva) with T-shaped symbols (movement), and a ram (strength and willpower).

- **Essential oils:** peppermint or clary sage to balance; juniper to cleanse.

- **Element:** sustained by the natural element of Fire.

- **Physical action:** major nerve plexus for the whole body.

- **Mental action:** empowerment or weakness of the ego; holds on to anxiety and fears.

- **Beneficial yoga asanas:** Ustrasana (camel), Uttana mayurasana (bridge).

This chakra is located within the aura below the sternum. The Sanskrit name for the Solar Plexus Chakra—meaning "jewel of the navel"—indicates that it is a treasure connecting us to solar consciousness.

This fiery chakra keeps us well by constantly bringing solar light-encoded energies into our body. They activate the great plexus (bundle) of nerves that radiate out from the physical solar plexus (in the pit of the stomach) like a sun, connecting to our metabolism and digestive processes. The specific glands that are stimulated are a group of cells called the Islets of Langerhans, which produce insulin within the pancreas. We could say that, in its own way, this chakra balances sweetness in our lives.

Physical disorders associated with an unbalanced Solar Plexus Chakra include muscular stiffness, stomach, digestive and liver problems, lower back pain, diabetes, hypoglycemia (low blood sugar), and fevers. This chakra helps to overcome nervous tension caused by stress. Rebalancing it is a major factor in increasing general bodily vitality and zest for life.

Balance the Solar Plexus Chakra

The Sun symbolizes the supreme cosmic power and potential within us all. The Solar Plexus Chakra is the fire center and hub of digestion, known in traditional Chinese medicine as the "triple warmer" because of the heat generated through processing and assimilating food. Poor digestion of food—or of ideas—is one of the first indications that the Solar Plexus Chakra is out of balance. Mostly this is because this chakra reacts to anxiety and fear, while key life issues revolve around emotional turmoil and materialism, which can in turn compromise physical health.

Through this chakra we can take on the thoughts and emotions of other people, or they can consciously (or unconsciously) withdraw energy from it, causing us to feel vulnerable. This may or may not be malicious, but it is vital for psychics and healers to protect the energies of their Solar Plexus Chakra.

Excessive energy can lead to becoming judgmental, a workaholic, a perfectionist, and resentful of authority.

Deficient energy signifies depression, insecurity, fear when alone, and poor digestion.

There are numerous ways to bring **balance** to this chakra and the essence is to reduce stress (*see* the following pages for some stress-reducing techniques). Although sometimes difficult, try to be cheerful, outgoing, relaxed, and uninhibited. When we are balanced, we show emotional warmth, enjoy good food, and physical activity.

Affirmation: "I honor the Sun as the source of life on Earth."

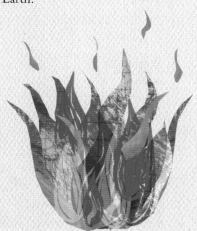

Stress Less

Stress is an attitude of mind that contributes to serious diseases, but people who regularly practice yoga and meditation have lowered stress levels and improved health, even at the level of their DNA.

Make a little special time for yourself each day, working with the following suggestions and activities. Learning to de-stress, before it chronically affects your body, is vital.

- Use a deep-breathing or body-relaxation technique, for all-over chakra balance.

- Review what is really important in your life, so that you don't overreact to petty events.

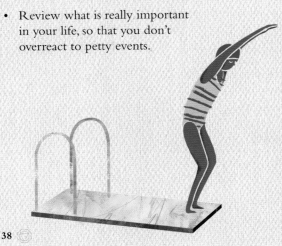

- Look after yourself and take time to do whatever you enjoy.

- Try practices such as yoga, Tai Chi, and Chi Kung, which harmonize energy flows. Tai Chi is traditionally practiced outdoors, for maximum benefit.

- Try out a new sport, as many sports aid relaxation.

- Being in nature—really tuning in to nature—is one of the best things you can do.

- Enjoy healthy relationships and loving sex.

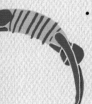

  - Explore the relaxing effects of crystals (*see* page 60) and essential oils (*see* page 82) for vaporizing or massage.

    - Immerse yourself in activities that feed your creativity, such as art, dance, or music.

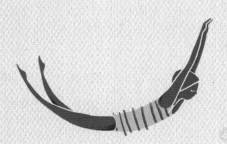

Activity: Sun Salutation —Surya Namaskara
(10 minutes)

This sequence of yoga asanas benefits all the chakras. Repeat it on each side of the body, creating flowing transitions between each position.

2 While inhaling, arch backward.

1 Start in a mountain pose (with your hands in prayer position), with normal, restful breathing while sensing revitalizing solar and pranic energy filling your body.

10 While exhaling, bring your feet together then stand up slowly, ready to start again.

9 While inhaling, step forward with right leg.

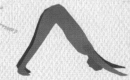

8 Exhale into inverted "V" position.

3 While exhaling, fold forward.

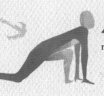

4 While inhaling, step back with right leg.

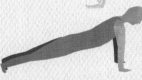

5 While exhaling, assume a straight body position, then pause breath.

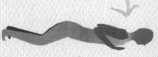

6 With breath still paused, slide onto your knees, chest, and chin.

7 While inhaling, slide into cobra pose.

Activity: Stress Busting
(10 minutes)

**If your solar plexus feels tight and knotted,
try the following moves.**

- Release stress in the solar plexus by massaging the
  area in a clockwise direction for a couple of minutes.

- Now stand up, take a very deep breath and release
  it forcefully through your mouth with a big, noisy
  sigh. Let all your stress go, using three or four of
  these breaths, then stand calmly.

- Breathe normally, smile to yourself, and swallow
  that smile. Yes, swallow it, with a little ball of saliva.
  Enjoy how that feels. A smile into your body
  recharges it, and you can then continue your day
  feeling much more relaxed. Swallowing your smile
  originates in Taoist meditation practice, Chi Kung,
  and internal martial arts.

4
Heart Chakra: Gentle Love

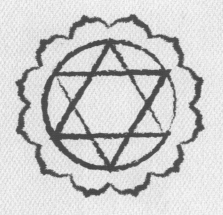

The Heart Chakra—Anahata

Well-being, gentle love, and unconditional relationships.

- **Traditional meaning:** the unstruck primordial sound; words on the 12 lotus petals represent negative traits that are destroyed by love.

- **Color:** resonates with soft, clear, green light frequencies.

- **Yantra:** two triangles forming a star shape, representing balance and harmony.

- **Essential oils:** neroli or rose for balance; thyme to cleanse.

- **Element:** sustained by the natural element of Air.

- **Physical action:** integrates complementary forces.

- **Mental action:** integrates the higher and lower nature.

- **Beneficial yoga asanas:** Bhujangasana (cobra), Janusirsasana (forward bend).

Located centrally within the aura near the heart, the Heart Chakra helps to keep us well by constantly bringing subtle pranic energy vibrations emanating from the green vegetation of the planet into our physical body. When this chakra develops into full bloom, its light frequencies gradually change to reflect the pink light of unconditional love.

The Heart Chakra is associated with the thymus—an organ that forms an important part of the body's immune defense system and is particularly vital in childhood.

Physical disorders can include high blood pressure, heart disease, lung disease, and asthma. Doctors now realize that stress plays a large part in heart health. From a chakra perspective, stresses concerned with romantic love and sexuality can become misplaced at the Heart Chakra instead of being resolved by the lower chakras. Such feelings can grow, putting strain on the physical heart, so that eventually our ability to love withers away. Increased awareness of our gentle love chakra helps to dispel these stresses.

Balance the Heart Chakra

Can you sense if this chakra is out of balance?
Perhaps you find deep relationships difficult,
you lack energy, or your heartbeat seems too fast
(if this is a recurring issue, consult your doctor)?

Excessive chakra energy can lead to being demanding,
overcritical, possessive, moody, and depressed, and to
giving love only with conditions imposed.

Deficient energy leads to indecisiveness, hanging on
to objects or people, fear of rejection, and the need for
constant reassurance. Key life-path issues are emotional
confusion, especially concerning relationships.

There are numerous ways to bring **balance:** by being
generous, compassionate, outgoing, friendly, and by
growing toward loving unconditionally. Great spiritual
teachers say that to "love ourselves" is a primary step
in awakening ourselves to higher consciousness. Unless
we have love and respect for ourselves, it is difficult
to extend the same feelings to others and our
relationships will suffer.

In our chakra exploration, the natural element of Air releases any excesses held at the heart that have not been dealt with by the lower chakras. So breathing deeply brings more pranic life force in: it revitalizes the bloodstream throughout our bodies. Deep breathing is a useful strategy because it immediately alleviates stress and contributes to feelings of well-being, which balance out relationship issues. In tense situations, try taking three deep breaths before speaking.

Affirmation: "Within my open heart lie the answers to all my questions."

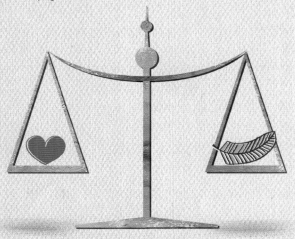

Activity: Being the Love
(10 minutes)

A simple strategy to cultivate unconditional love is to imagine yourself in another person's place. What would your wants and needs be then? Reflecting upon this lets the Heart Chakra blossom, because the symbolic lotus petals unfold to receive even more love and light. Not only does this nourish another person or creature, but it also nourishes you at a profound spiritual level.

Try this meditation to open the petals of the heart.

- Sit comfortably and close your eyes. Breathe deeply three times.

- **Imagine:** "I am sitting in a forest with my back against a tree. Becoming one with the rich green of the tree's leaves, I breathe this color into my lungs and heart. Exhaling, I let the green breath take any emotional pain from my heart back into the Earth.

"Now I see a perfect pink lotus bud in a still pool of water. I find I can open up many of the petals, for I know each one represents something that I now need to release. Finally, I increase my radiance with a loving burst of golden light directed to myself and others."

• Resolve to continue this meditation on other days, until the lotus is fully open, your heart is cleared of past traumas, and compassion becomes your "default" mode.

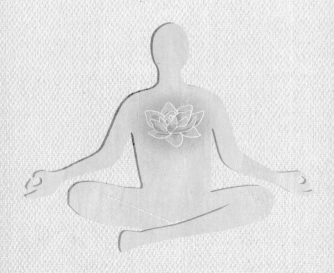

Activity: Pendulum Power
(10 minutes)

You can discover your chakra balance using
a pendulum, although it takes a while to build
up empathy with your pendulum. If it is a crystal,
cleanse it first (*see* page 61). When using a crystal
pendulum, never hold it directly over a chakra
or it will immediately stimulate it—instead, hold
one hand over the chakra and the other hand
(the one holding the pendulum) away to the side.

- Establish the direction in which your pendulum
  moves, by asking questions to which the answer is
  "Yes". For example, "Is it Tuesday [or whatever the
  correct day is] today?" Note the pendulum's response.

- Find your pendulum's "No" response by asking
  a silly question that is untrue, such as "Am I a horse?"
  Keep going with "Yes" and "No" questions until
  the pendulum's reaction is reliable. Eventually it
  will always turn in a particular direction for "Yes"
  and in the opposite direction for "No".

- Now check your chakras: feeling relaxed, with
  a still mind and feeling unattached to the result,

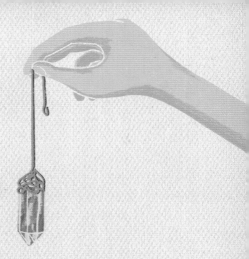

hold the pendulum by a chakra and ask questions such as "Is this chakra overactive?" and "Is this chakra underactive?" As your pendulum responds, make a chart of the results and date it.

- Once you have ascertained an imbalance in a specific chakra with the help of a pendulum, you can practice any of the appropriate self-healing techniques for that chakra as described in this book. Then use the pendulum again to check it is balanced. Alternatively, you may wish to seek the assistance of an accredited chakra healer.

Count Your Blessings

**Ask yourself the following questions and note
your answers.**

- How many good things have I been given today?

- What have I given to others?

- Have I been grateful?

- When might I have been unnecessarily judgmental?

- How many smiles have I given to others?

- Did I scowl or use hurtful words?

- Just how many blessings did I receive today?

- And how many did I give?

Lao-Tzu, the 6th-century B.C.E. Chinese philosopher, said:

> ## Without leaving his house,
> ## one can know everything
> ## that is necessary.
>
> ## Without leaving himself
> ## one can grasp all wisdom.

5
Throat Chakra:
Sound

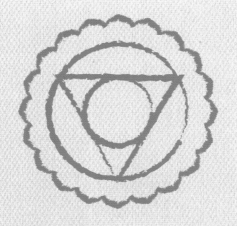

The Throat Chakra—Vishuddha

Breath, sound, and harmony.

- **Traditional meaning:** to purify; the 16 lotus petals have Sanskrit letters.

- **Color:** resonates with pale or turquoise-blue light frequencies.

- **Yantra:** 16 lotus petals, silver crescent (purity and sacred sound), downward-pointing yellow triangle (energy of Akasha or Ether) in a white circle (moon and psychic powers), and a white elephant who carries the sound mantra.

- **Essential oils:** lavender or chamomile to balance; rosemary to cleanse.

- **Element:** sustained by the natural element of Ether or Akasha, meaning the essence of infinite space, sky, or atmosphere.

- **Physical action:** purifies the body.

- **Mental action:** purifies the mind.

- **Beneficial yoga asanas:**
  Paschimottanasana
  (forward bend),
  Matsyasana (fish).

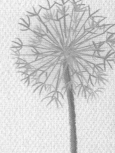

Located within the aura at the throat, the Throat Chakra helps to keep us well by constantly bringing subtle energy vibrations from the Earth's atmosphere and sky into our physical body. In yogic traditions this is the refined Air element of Ether or Akasha. This chakra is a "bridge" between higher and lower states of being and its main task is to absorb and purify, in the elevated realm of Ether or Akasha, the other natural elements of Earth, Water, Fire, and Air.

This chakra center is closely associated with the respiratory system as well as the thyroid and parathyroid glands, which bring equilibrium to the body's systems. Physical disorders arising from imbalance include exhaustion, body weight being too high or low, thyroid, neck, and throat problems, and neck and head pain.

When you are centered at the Throat Chakra, you connect with deeper levels of the mind. This process is traditionally enhanced by breathing exercises (called "Pranayama" in yoga), the chanting of prayers, or the repetition and intoning of the sacred sounds known as "mantras" (*see* page 58).

Balance the Throat Chakra

One of the ways that the Throat Chakra purifies and assists in the development of meditation and spiritual wisdom is through "Satya," a Sanskrit word for truthfulness of speech and actions, being the second of the yogic "Yamas" or virtuous restraints. Mindfulness and truthfulness enable us to speak our deepest desires; in contrast, if we lie to ourselves—or others—we become vulnerable.

Excessive energy can lead to becoming over-stimulated, arrogant, dogmatic, and talking excessively.

Deficient energy means being overfearful, inconsistent, unreliable, manipulative, and avoiding sex.

Key life-path issues concern shallow breathing and poor communication. Yogic breathing (Pranayama) brings **balance**, making us feel centered within and helping us to be a good speaker, artist, singer, or instrumentalist. Learning honest, clear communication and how to express ourselves through song are the gifts and blessings of this chakra.

To work deeply with our sound chakra, we need to tune into the subtle vibrational fields around us in the natural world. The sounds of nature are music for the soul.

- Take time out from a busy life to sit still; you don't even have to be alone. Some may call this daydreaming.

- Close your eyes. Listen to the sounds around you, and notice ones that are disharmonious and those that have a natural harmony and are relaxing and nourishing. Sounds can either be a "food" or a pollutant.

Affirmation: "I communicate with clarity and sing with passion."

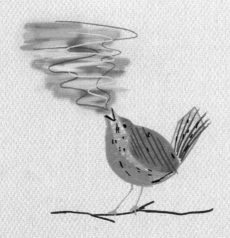

Mantras

Om mani padme hum.
(God is a precious jewel
in the lotus of my heart)

A traditional Tibetan mantra.

**Mantras are repetitive incantations or prayers
stemming from Hinduism and other religious
practices. The word "mantra" means "the thought
that liberates and protects" and reciting mantras
unlocks the ability to deepen your relaxation and
change your consciousness.**

Sound therapy demonstrates that all sounds—including
everyday language and the sounds of nature—create
beneficial or detrimental vibrational frequencies. Some
frequencies are above, and others are below, our ability
to hear. Sounds ripple through air, water, and solids,
charging a vast electromagnetic field, which is part
of the Web of Life (*see* page 70).

Practicing mantras ideally takes place alongside Pranayama
breath-control techniques or as a centering method
before meditation.

Activity: Toning (10 minutes)

Here are the traditional sound-tones known as "bija" (or "little jewel") mantras associated with each chakra, which are easy to say out loud. Practice repeating the bija mantra for each individual chakra a number of times. Then go through them sequentially, from the Base Chakra up to the Crown Chakra, before returning back down to the Base Chakra again.

Base Chakra: Lam (*lahm*)

Sacral Chakra: Vam (*vahm*)

Solar Plexus Chakra: Ram (*rahm*)

Heart Chakra: Yam (*yahm*)

Throat Chakra: Ham (*hahm*)

Brow Chakra: Ksham (*k'shahm*)

Crown Chakra: Om (*ah-oh-mmm*)

Balancing the Chakras with Crystals

Crystals can be used in various ways to balance the life-force that flows through the chakras. Certain crystals have an affinity with particular chakras, as shown below, so choose a crystal that relates to the specific chakra you wish to work on.

Base Chakra: carnelian or obsidian.

Sacral Chakra: moonstone or aquamarine.

Solar Plexus Chakra: citrine or clear quartz.

Heart Chakra: rose quartz or green aventurine.

Throat Chakra: turquoise or chrysocolla.

Brow Chakra: lapis lazuli or sapphire.

Crown Chakra: amethyst or clear quartz.

For the three celestial chakras, *see* page 90 onward.

How to cleanse and use crystals

Cleanse your crystal's auric field by washing it in pure water, then drying it in sunlight. You are now ready either to hold your crystal in your hand during meditation or to place it on, or close to, the chakra that you have chosen to work on. Be kind to yourself and balance one chakra at a time, so that you can sense and memorize the effect it has.

Complete chakra boost

You can boost all the chakras using two quartz crystals with single points.

- Lie down on your back and place one large quartz crystal on the floor with its point facing toward your head, and the other crystal just below your feet, pointing centrally up your body. These crystals are highly directional, so they will boost the whole seven-chakra system.

- You need only relax. The crystals and spirit will do whatever balancing is required.

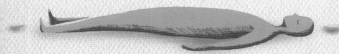

Activity: Sounding "OM"
(10 minutes)

Now is the time to experiment with your voice. Don't be afraid to express yourself. Sounding "OM" aids relaxation and charges your lungs with pranic energy. This is beneficial to your whole body, bringing you into a state of "being," not "doing."

- Either stand or sit with a straight spine, having ensured that you will not be disturbed.

- Become aware of your inner peace and inhale deeply; then slowly release the sounds as you exhale, stretching your mouth and jaw muscles: "OM" is sounded like "A-U-M," in three parts, making one continuous sound: "Ahhhhh, Ohhhh, Mmmm," Notice how the sound moves from the back of your throat to the front of your mouth.

- Strengthen the experience by repeating "OM" six or nine times. (Meditation is enhanced by chanting "OM" at the beginning and end of the session.)

- Remember to enjoy the silence between each "OM." Don't hurry.

6
Brow Chakra:
Insight

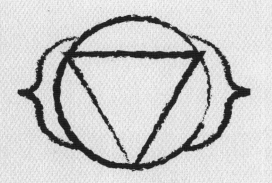

The Brow Chakra—Ajna

Inner sight, intuition, harmony with nature.

- **Traditional meaning**: to know; the two open lotus petals represent balance of opposites, including left and right hemispheres of the brain.

- **Color**: resonates with deep-blue frequencies of light.

- **Yantra**: an inverted triangle, representing reality, consciousness and joy ("sat," "chit," "ananda").

- **Essential oils**: frankincense to balance; holy basil to cleanse.

- **Element**: sustained by the natural element of Ether or Akasha, meaning the essence of infinite space, sky, or atmosphere.

- **Physical action**: brings equilibrium to the brain.

- **Mental action**: balances ego and the higher consciousness.

- **Beneficial yoga asanas**: Nataraja asana (dancer), Garudasana (eagle).

Located within the aura near the middle of the brow, our Brow (or Insight) Chakra, among other functions,

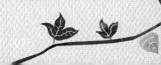

balances the circadian rhythms of sleeping and waking. To do this it brings subtle energetic vibrations of Ether or Akasha—such as those from the night sky—into our physical body through the pituitary gland. It is traditionally associated with a minor chakra (*see* page 8) known as Soma (or "amrit," meaning Divine Nectar of Life), from which this fluid is said to flow.

Also called our "Third Eye," the Brow Chakra is closely associated with the pituitary gland, eyes, ears, nose, nervous system, and the brain. Physical disorders associated with it include headaches, some eye and sinus problems, sleeplessness, and hormonal imbalances. Balancing everyday activities is one of the main roles of this chakra, so we should ideally have sound sleep, healthy food, time for relaxation, a fulfilling working life, and good relationships. Inwardly we meld developing insights with wisdom, to express joy and positivity.

Key life-path issues are overstimulation of psychic powers, leading to control over others.

Balance the Brow Chakra

Many branches of yoga teach that this insight chakra should be stimulated and opened gradually, with a balance of the lower chakras being a prerequisite otherwise disorientation can result. This is the chakra where two streams of life energy channels, called the Ida and Pingala, meet and terminate, joining with the central energy channel, Sushumna. Esoterically, this action is connected to the rising of Kundalini (*see* page 28) and to the symbolic sexual union of god and goddess.

Our consciousness expands from this chakra; we become unattached to material possessions, fame, or fortune and have no fear of death.

Excessive energy can lead to being religiously dogmatic, overly proud and manipulative, and susceptible to the inappropriate force of ego.

Deficient energy means being oversensitive, nonassertive, and unable to distinguish between your ego and your true higher self.

There are numerous ways to bring **balance** to mind and body. More than any other chakra, working on your Brow Chakra unlocks insights and develops latent psychic powers of telepathy, clairaudience (super-sensory hearing), clairvoyance (super-sensory insight), and access to past lives. Naturally, these powers need to be used positively and wisely, for we can so easily, and unthinkingly, slip back into imbalance.

Affirmation: "My inner eye reflects my inner Light."

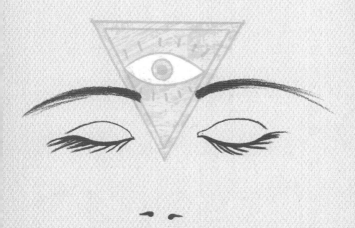

Activity: Concentrate on a Candle Flame (10 minutes)

By concentrating your focus on a candle flame you can boost the Brow Chakra.

- Sit comfortably in simple crossed-leg position (Sukhasana) or on a straight-backed chair. Alternatively, take another yoga sitting position, such as the lotus position (Padmasana) or half-lotus (Siddhasana).

- Light a candle, placing it about 18 inches in front of you. Be still and look at the flame without blinking, and with complete attention, for a few minutes.

- Close your eyes and watch the residual image that appears at the center of your brow, until it disappears.

- Open your eyes and either repeat the activity or blink a few times.

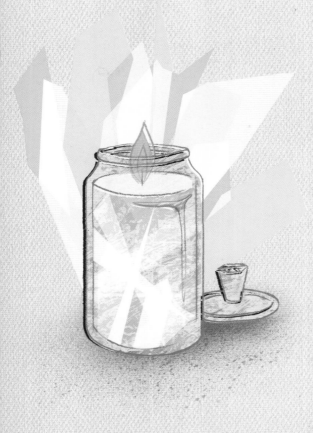

Being in Nature

The Web of Life embodies the time-honored idea that all life forms are related and interdependent. Present-day science calls this the Morphogenetic Field, or just "the Field." Its unseen energy (including prana) surrounds and interpenetrates us in a multidimensional way, filtering into our body cells and passing messages to them. Messages from a polluted environment can harm us, but we receive the gift of healthy encodements from the Web of Life through the Base Chakra, the Earth Star Chakra (*see* page 86), and all the other chakras, to help our body function.

Being outside in nature and opening up to this positive web recharges body, mind, and spirit; the prana in a flowing stream nourishes the Water element of our bodies, and sunshine activates the inner Fire of our metabolism.

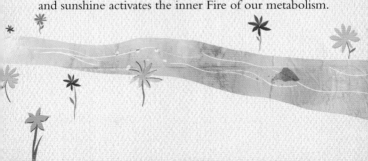

Activity: Recharging Relaxation
(10 minutes)

Recharge the Brow Chakra using this soothing relaxation technique. If you have a dysfunction or disease in your body, it is particularly useful to visualize this, because your body knows how to restore itself. As a part of nature, your cellular organism is always striving for equilibrium and the healthiest possible options.

- Lie on your back in the yoga relaxation asana known as Savasana—outside, if possible.

- **Imagine:** "I connect to the Web of Life, imagining waves of light first penetrating my aura, then my chakras. Instantaneously, deep within me, bursts of life-sustaining light activate every cell in my body. This happens constantly, but my 'superconscious' awareness enhances it."

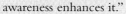

Activity: Recharge with Sun Energies (5 minutes)

This activity prepares you to access your higher chakras. If you can be outside, sitting in a simple crossed-leg position (Sukhasana), this is ideal. You will still benefit from this visualization if you are at your office desk or taking a short break from your daily routine.

- Let your eyes close gently and feel your breath flowing through your nose into your lungs.

- **Imagine:** "I can visualize a vibrant golden ball of sunlight filling my solar plexus region. Shafts of light infuse and energize my whole body. If any part is in discomfort, I will direct this golden healing light to that place."

- At the end of the visualization, contemplate how you feel.

7
Crown Chakra: Spirit

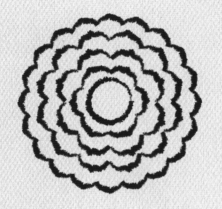

The Crown Chakra—Sahasrara

Reaching higher illumination and spirit.

- **Traditional meaning:** one thousandfold; the petals represent pure consciousness.

- **Color:** resonates with violet, gold, and white light frequencies.

- **Yantra:** 1,000 lotus petals (Divine knowledge), upward-pointing yellow triangle (spiritual Sun) with crescent moon (duality transformed), and a supreme bindu (dot symbolizing supreme silence attained by sounding "OM").

- **Essential oils:** linden or lotus to balance spiritual energies.

- **Element:** sustained by Spirit.

- **Physical action:** refines the brain and nervous system.

- **Mental action:** inner understanding or enlightenment.

- **Beneficial yoga asanas:** Sirasana (headstand) or simple head-down positions.

Located within the aura just above the head, the Crown Chakra of the thousand-petaled lotus is the final destination of kundalini (*see* page 28) and has numerous

specialized meanings. When kundalini reaches this
chakra, it no longer belongs to the realms of human
awareness; it is purely Divine—energy and consciousness
unite and illumination dawns. Together with the Brow
Chakra, the Crown Chakra pulses these forces down
through the central spiritual channel, the Sushumna,
enabling you to sense bliss. However, key life-path
issues about conforming within society may challenge
true enlightenment. It's not so easy for us to live
a devotional life or spend years in spiritual retreat.

The endocrine glands associated with this chakra are
the pineal and pituitary glands, which keep the body
in equilibrium. Physical disorders include brain disease,
disorders of the endocrine system, and deeply disturbing
psychological problems—the last possibly associated
with past Karma (*see* page 91).

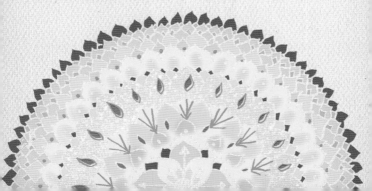

Balance the Crown Chakra

Our Crown Chakra resonates with the clear white light of spirit. It helps to keep us well by constantly making subtle energy vibrations available to our physical body. Without this chakra transmuting and stepping down these vibrations, we would not be able to absorb them.

Excessive energy can lead to frustration, frequent migraines, and restlessness, showing that we are overloading this chakra, perhaps, in a spiritual sense, by not putting in the groundwork and trying to run before we can walk, for instance, persistently attempting to attain psychic powers. Sometimes this spirit chakra activates before we are ready to cope with it; maybe we have experimented with drugs or have opened ourselves up to dubious powers. In these instances the Crown Chakra can spin too fast or be erratic, or it may be permanently wedged "open." Careful balancing of all the chakras by a dedicated healer is recommended.

Deficient energy signifies indecision and a lack of joy in life.

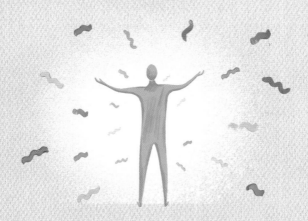

There are numerous tools and ways to bring about **balance** described in this book, and a positive mind is the key. When you are balanced, you become open to Divine radiance and super-consciousness while in your normal awakened state. Initially you may only experience these higher states for a short time, as a burst of indescribable bliss. However, activating mindfulness while living a compassionate "Path of Light" means that you will learn to tune into them ecstatically.

Affirmation: "Whenever I choose goodness and wisdom, I open to my full potential."

Activity: Protecting Subtle Energies (5 minutes)

As you reach different levels of chakra perception, you need to nurture and protect your understanding of it against any leaking of energy. This can be done in several ways.

- Realizing that your insights are your own inner truths, and not talking excessively about them or being egotistical.

- Placing a "cloak of protection" around your auric field, by imagining wrapping yourself totally in a deep-blue velvet cloak.

- Creating a protective sphere of light around yourself. You can do this in an instant: imagine that you are sending light from your right hand spinning around your body. Then extend this light-shield into a sphere or egg shape around yourself, extending as far out as the distance you can stretch your arms. This is sometimes called "egging up."

Now you are protected from any leakage of subtle energies through your aura, for even among those who seem well intentioned, there are people who will drain your energy; sometimes you can just feel it. Then there are those who will question you constantly about what you are doing—not wanting to do the hard work themselves—and in the process will try to steal your spiritual gold. They are jokingly called "energy vampires."

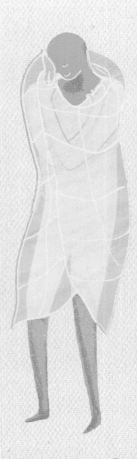

Energy and Prana

Breathing in prana (the life force) is one way
to increase its power within you, connecting
you to the Web of Life (*see* page 70).
Together, Earth-consciousness—born from
an understanding that the planet is a living
entity—and pranic energy show the way
to infinite peace. You will then find yourself
immersed in an outpouring of Divine Light.

Here are two ways to help you understand how
energy flows through your higher chakras.

- Nature's gift of crystals can alter your physical rate
  of vibration. For instance, celestite (a powerful
  pale-blue crystal) activates the Crown Chakra,
  enabling the perception of other realms. Sit quietly
  and meditate with this crystal and see what is revealed.

- Alternatively, you can be active and can tune into
  your chakras through music, movement, and dance
  (*see* opposite).

Free Expression with Dance

Although musical taste is a very personal thing, a piece of harmonious, inspirational music may tempt you to try the following.

- Play your chosen music. Stand, poised and still, breathing gently.

- Begin moving with the music, experiencing the exhilaration of spinning or stillness, movement and stretching. Dance freely to awaken your inner being. Be aware of how the pulse of the music lets you free up your body, so that you move in all of the available space.

- Eventually the music will take your dance to a conclusion and you will naturally want to lie down for a few moments. Note how your chakras feel recharged and harmonized.

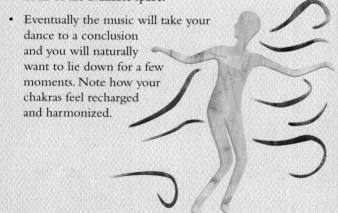

Using Essential Plant Oils

**The pure essential oils used in aromatherapy
represent the highest vibration of plant energies—
more powerful than the growing plants or the
medicinal herbs themselves. Using essential oils,
you can easily tune into the life force energies of
the plant, and such oils are extremely compatible
with expanded human consciousness. Due to their
potency, however, it is important to use them wisely.**

Essential oils may be vaporized with water, to create
a beneficial fragrance in a room; alternatively, a few
drops of essential oil in bathwater can be calming. Select
the appropriate balancing oil for the chakra in question
(from the list in the introduction to each chakra in this
book) and spend ten minutes breathing in the fragrance.
You might prefer to use essential oils for a massage, in which
case dilute them before use with a bland "carrier" oil, such
as almond or grapeseed, in the proportions of two teaspoons
of carrier oil to a maximum of five drops of essential oil.

*Note: There are no oils listed for the newly emerging chakras on the following
pages because they relate to Spirit rather than the body and natural remedies.*

8
Newly Emerging Chakras

New Awareness

Historically, the seven traditional chakras have sustained humanity. But now, as the whole of human consciousness is poised to make momentous decisions—whether to transform as a global family or head the way of the dinosaurs—significant evolutionary energies are flooding into our planetary field, prompting us to act. Should we choose to evolve (and this does not even have to be a conscious decision), we will bring newly emerging chakras "on-stream."

These chakras lie both within and beyond the aura: one beneath the feet; another boosting the Sacral Chakra; and three celestial chakras in vertical alignment above the head. Each has special quantum qualities and transmits or receives multidimensional enlightenment codes to and from all the other chakras. The modern symbols for them reflect their color, energy, and spiritual qualities.

Humanity is currently in survival mode, shedding old ways based on thought patterns and actions that are rooted in the past. We are gradually discovering a new

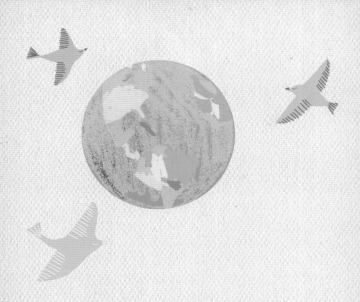

way of being, with compassion, integrity, and openness. Despite challenges caused by fear, stress, and grief, there is a way to find the inner peace that we crave. By going within, for just ten minutes—or with regular practice of relaxation or a deep-breathing technique, as taught in this book—you can alleviate the worst moments in your day. You will find a way to get through and, in the process, will become grounded and strong, like a mighty tree.

The Earth Star Chakra

A newly emerging chakra, located beneath the feet.

- **Color:** light is absent when dormant, changing to magenta light frequencies when awakened.

- **Crystal:** black obsidian to ground energies.

- **Energy:** sustained by beneficial flowing energies from the Earth.

- **Physical action:** grounds chakra energies deep into the Earth beneath.

- **Mental action:** awakens profound environmental awareness.

- **Beneficial yoga asana:** Savasana (relaxation pose).

The Earth Star Chakra is awakening. It complements the Base Chakra, being the prime grounding location for more refined vibrations that are descending from higher chakras, transferred through the legs and feet into the Earth Star. The influx of these supercharged energies causes this chakra to expand. It is dull when dormant, but awakens—shining with magenta-colored light—like a star beneath our feet. The Earth Star Chakra then deeply

roots us in our natural environment, while charging
it with light and great spirit wherever we tread.

In this way the Earth Star becomes a super, high-potential
chakra for our present times, when the Earth is so in need
of positive action. As our ecological awareness deepens,
we wake up to an unstoppable pulse of change. By
reprogramming new responses and by grounding high-
frequency "messages" in our immediate environment, we
can bring about far-reaching effects on the greater whole.

Forest bathing:

Imagine, as you walk, that the Earth Star Chakra is
always beneath your feet. Or experience the Japanese
way of immersing your senses in nature—called Shinrin
Yoku or "forest bathing"—in which you walk and relax
in the forest, developing mindfulness or meditation while
deeply breathing in the natural elements and tree essences
around you.

Affirmation: "I open to the great mystery of life."

The Hara Chakra

The root of vital life-force energy.

- **Color:** resonates with orange-yellow light frequencies.

- **Crystal:** carnelian to balance.

- **Energy:** the root and origin of Ki vital energy (*see* below).

- **Physical action:** distributes Ki around the body.

- **Mental action:** overcomes fears.

- **Beneficial yoga asanas:** Salabhasana (locust), Uddiyana (abdominal lift).

The Hara (meaning "belly") Chakra is another newly developing chakra to awaken, located within the auric field just above the Sacral Chakra. It connects us to wisdom of the East and becomes active in people who practice Eastern martial arts and energy techniques. In Oriental medicine, the hara is the root of vital energy, a dynamic part of the meridian energy channels that circulate around Ki (or Qi, pronounced "chee")—vital

life-force energy. In this system of medicine,
a stable hara and robust health go hand-in-hand.

Yoga teaches that all the energy channels (nadis)
originate from the navel as the source of life. If you
have not worked with your own fears, passions, and
pleasures and are not grounded (aspects of the Base
and Sacral Chakras), then it is difficult to awaken the
Hara Chakra.

The Hara, Heart, and Crown Chakras are the symbolic
Three Diamonds in the mastership of Reiki healing.
Key life-path issues question whether you should
expend energy on worthless pursuits and whether
you use subtle energy wisely.

Focus and inwardly ask yourself:

Is my hara active, the core of my body strong, my muscles
functioning optimally and my body systems resilient?

Affirmation: "I realize that all is energy."

The Causal Chakra

The first of the celestial chakras.

- **Color:** resonates with aqua light frequencies.

- **Crystal:** clear quartz or Herkimer diamond to increase awareness of this chakra.

- **Energy:** exchanges energy with the guiding higher consciousness.

- **Physical action:** prompts the body to act.

- **Mental action:** channels guidance.

- **Beneficial yoga asana:** Tadasana (mountain).

We begin unpacking the three celestial chakras with the Causal Chakra vortex, our connection with the Solar System, positioned some 4 inches above the Crown Chakra. Each of the celestial chakras is transpersonal in nature, so even though the Causal Chakra is not associated with the body, essential life guidance is received through this chakra during meditation and while you are experiencing silent peace. This is the chakra that causes—or guides—momentous occurrences in our lives, but this only arises in an ego-less space, in unity with our highest aspirations.

Through the Causal Chakra we might attain awareness of our "soul groups," which may (or may not) be in physical incarnation—they may be in other dimensions. In our present lives, this chakra is closely connected to the accumulation of Earth-bound "Karma": the spiritual law of cause-and-effect, and a kind of psychic baggage that we have chosen to carry—or release. With an active Causal Chakra, and as evolutionary pioneers of new consciousness, we are poised to journey onward, free of earthly pain and suffering.

Using crystals with the Causal Chakra:

- Cleanse your crystals before use (*see* page 61).

- Sit comfortably in a simple crossed-leg position (Sukhasana).

- Holding your chosen crystal, enter into a deep meditative state.

- To balance the Causal Chakra hold moonstone or celestite. To direct healing to the Causal Chakra, lie on your back and place a kyanite crystal pointing toward the top of your head.

Affirmation: "I release all that is not needed and cherish my insights."

The Soul Star Chakra

The second of the celestial chakras.

- **Color:** resonates with peach–pink light frequencies.

- **Crystal:** pink petalite or pink opal to increase awareness of this chakra.

- **Energy:** aligned with personal and planetary healing.

- **Physical action:** stimulates DNA codes or functions.

- **Mental action:** opens to spirit and transcendental consciousness.

- **Beneficial yoga practices:** Surya kumbhaka (alternate nostril-breathing) and regular meditation.

The Soul Star Chakra vortex is located around 6 inches above the Crown Chakra. It connects with the Milky Way galaxy, which transmits energies to and from an awakened individual. Some people are blessed with the gifts of healing and channeling Divine Light energies that originate in the beyond; they are aligned at this chakra. All higher chakras are receptive to crystals, and healers sometimes use pink petalite or a rod of selenite crystal to increase light vibrations.

Although it is unconnected to specific physical body systems, this chakra may be involved in stimulating DNA life codes, through unidentified quantum energies that work in a multidimensional way.

Most importantly, immediately after the death of the body, the Soul Star Chakra is the abode of the soul. In this process of release from the Earth, a trained healer may assist during the soul's departure.

Activating the Soul Star:

• Sit comfortably in a simple crossed-leg position (Sukhasana) or the lotus position (Padmasana).

• Focus on how, when the traditional seven chakras are in harmony, activation of the Soul Star Chakra is possible during deep introspection or mindful meditation.

Affirmation: "My life journey is but a beginning."

The Stellar Gateway

The third of the celestial chakras.

- **Color:** resonates with sparkling clear, white light.

- **Crystal:** green moldavite crystal to increase awareness of this chakra.

- **Energy:** our primary connection to other realms.

- **Physical action:** calms through meditation.

- **Mental action:** brings Quantum Consciousness (*see* opposite).

- **Beneficial yoga practice:** regular prolonged meditation.

The Stellar Gateway is our connection with the universe and other realms of being, after we leave our body. It is multidimensional, holographic, interstellar, and timeless. With the other celestial chakras, it assists the tender, beneficial evolution of all humanity, as we face unprecedented changes on Earth.

During life, this vortex is located 12 inches above the Crown Chakra, but—like the other celestial chakras—

its position varies enormously, and it may be way beyond our physical body in the wider light-energy field. When it is aligned with the higher intentions of other chakras (and if a person's soul-path requires it), this chakra brings Quantum Consciousness—a type of consciousness that takes us simultaneously both within and beyond our normal understandings. Deep introspection and meditation help us to contemplate this chakra's gifts.

Opening the Stellar Gateway:

- Sit peacefully and breathe deeply.
- During meditation, hold a piece of moldavite, a clear green crystal of extraterrestrial origin, which helps to activate and prime the opening of the Stellar Gateway Chakra. Sense how this chakra refines your choices and holds your challenges as if in a loving embrace.

Affirmation: "As I strive for balance and wellness, I know my journey's end is beyond the stars."

Acknowledgments

To Michael, the dreamer and my life's muse.

Immense gratitude to: the wonder and mystery of the natural world that supports and enables me to touch into the energetic nature of the universe; the many wise teachers I have met during my life journey, notably Barbara Griggs my very first Yoga teacher who "opened my eyes"; my esoteric master who preferred his famous name to be hidden; Theo Gimbel, inspirational color and light healing pioneer; the books of eminent Dr. Ervin Laszlo, a "cutting-edge" philosopher, evolution theorist, and visionary author; Maya elders Hunbatz Men and "Tata" Don Alejandro Cirilo Perez Oxlaj who shared their ceremonies and ancient star-born wisdom with me in those magical lands of the Maya peoples, Central America.

Acknowledging, of course, the brilliant editors, illustrator, and design and production teams at Gaia, Octopus Publishing Group, who brought this delightful book to fruition. I hope you have enjoyed reading it as much as I have enjoyed writing it!